Persistent Postural-Perceptual Dizziness (PPPD) Remedy Guide:

Detailed Guide on Persistent Postural-Perceptual Dizziness (PPPD); Causes & Signs; Efficient Treatment; Physical Therapy & Lots More

By

Doctor Peter L. Turnbull

Copyright@2021

TABLE OF CONTENTS

CHAPTER 1

INTRODUCTION

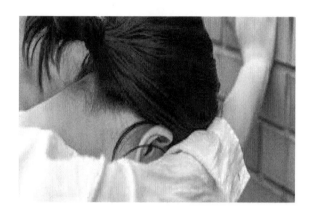

Persistent postural-
perceptual dizziness (PPPD)
otherwise called Chronic
abstract discombobulation
(CSD) is a condition where
patients experience a

steady impression of tipsiness for example dazedness the entire day, consistently. Normally patients are touchy to head developments or development of their environmental factors. In the event that patients become bleary eyed when there is development of their environmental elements or when the visual climate is occupied for example in a store, the mark "visual dizziness" is likewise utilized. Normally patients feel better when they are not moving.

On the off chance that no other reason is found for the discombobulation and the patient has a sensation of insecurity which is more regrettable with head development, development of their environmental elements or occupied visual climate, then, at that point, PPPD is a potential mark which could be applied to their condition. The specific reason for this issue is hazy yet in certain patients there is an unmistakable hastening occasion like BPPV, vestibular neuronitis (viral labyrinthitis), headache, head or neck injury or a scene of wretchedness/mental pressure.

The next chapters reveal all you need to know concerning

Persistent postural-

perceptual dizziness (PPPD)

from a to z.

CHAPTER 2

CAUSES, MANAGEMENT, POTENTIAL TRIGGERS, PHYSICAL THERAPY AND TREATMENT

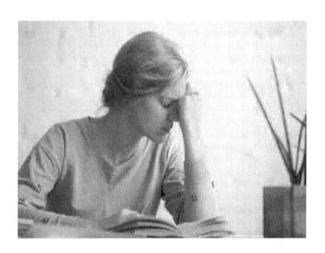

Different reasons for persistent unsteadiness

Patient with Multi-factorial unsteadiness can likewise have relentless tipsiness. Patient with multifactorial dazedness as a rule have numerous other ailments (diabetes, joint issues, nerve/neurological issues, visual issues or are on various different meds). Patient with respective vestibular hypofunction can likewise feel woozy while preparing however they tend not have affectability to a visual climate. They regularly portray precariousness. While sitting in a seat they can shake their head from one side to another fast without it having an enduring wooziness.

In PPPD it is especially significant that patients are evaluated by their GP for conditions other than ear illness which might be causing discombobulation. This incorporates low circulatory strain, unpredictable heart beat (arrhythmia), sickliness (low blood count), unusual degrees of salts or sugar in the blood, strange chemicals (for example low Thyroid chemical), low Vitamin levels (for example Nutrient D or B12), irritation in or around the mind, unusual capacity of nerves.

The Management One Should Know

There is anything but a solitary and generally concurred treatment. Extensively the medicines incorporate desensitization/remuneration and medication treatment (or both).

Visual/vestibular desensitization/remuneratio

n. This includes continuously expanding openness to the circumstances that can make dazedness in an endeavour develop your resistance. For instance, a few patients feel bleary eyed especially when going to the general store, driving or in any event, strolling outside for example in swarms. The movement/exercise should endure somewhere around a couple of moments and be adequately quick to cause some wooziness/repulsiveness for a couple of moments after you stop. This permits the mind to either adjust as well as redress. Sadly, numerous patients with CSD are delicate to any boosts (regardless of whether activities or medication treatment) and acclimate/repay gradually. After an activity you should intend to keep this time of "repulsiveness" to beneath thirty minutes if conceivable. This would permit you to rehash the activity 2 to 3 times each day. On the off chance that the period repulsiveness keeps going longer than 30 minutes it is probably going to exasperate the general issue. Whenever required you would have to lessen the intricacy, speed and length of movement. Obviously, you do need to complete the action for a couple of moments in any case no advantage/progress will be made. You might select to complete the action for a more limited term however more oftentimes for instance brief 5 times each day as opposed to 5 minutes 3 times each day. You should choose yourself if the action is sensible.

In the event that developments of your encompassing hasten the tipsiness in any event, when your head is still, then, at that point, the "disco ball" work out (optokinetic incitement) might be of some advantage. This includes sitting in a totally dull room with a rack behind you at a similar level as the highest point of your head. On the rack place a youngsters' disco ball (this can be bought from the kids' segment of shops like Argos or Amazon) which discharges moving example of kaleidoscopic lights onto the dividers. As referenced above, increment your openness slowly so the activity causes some disagreeableness which goes on for not exactly thirty minutes. This should be carried 3 times each day over half a month. In the event that you discover you can't endure any huge timeframe with the disco ball practice you might select to permit some light into the room at first.

When you are certain about your own home you can advance to practices outside. In the event that you can't endure strolling great, start with a short stroll to the furthest limit of your own way. Continuously increment the time of strolling or driving. You might wish to stroll in jam-packed regions at first toward the group and later the other way. Regarding stores which are regularly a reason for issues for patients I would suggest a short visit at first with the point of not really doing any shopping for example simply strolling through the paths. The fixation needed to keep up with your equilibrium and searching for explicit things for your shopping may at first be excessively difficult. Progressively as you can stroll around for longer periods you would then be able to start to really search for things. At first you might expect to buy things whose position/place is known to you.

A few patients appear to be narrow minded to the lights in grocery stores or are experience issues seeing things on a PC or in any event, perusing a book. I would suggest utilizing shades or coloured overlays which can be put over a PC screen or book. Coloured overlays can be bought from shops selling material for youngsters with dyslexia.

Treatment; More Explanations

Treatment is pointed toward aiding the cerebrum restoration with a superior feeling of insight and equilibrium. This is improved by utilizing exercise-based recuperation, prescriptions that work on serotonin levels in the cerebrum and now and again mental treatment to assist with decreasing the tension related with this upsetting condition. Most patients seek some help with the medicines, yet some can have manifestations for all time.

Potential Triggers

The specific reason for PPPD isn't yet known. Be that as it may, it frequently begins after one of these issues:

A vestibular or equilibrium problem that influences the internal ear or cerebrum.

Vestibular headache – a kind of headache involving cerebral pain that causes dizziness or tipsiness.

Tension that causes discombobulation or wooziness.

A blackout

Autonomic issues that cause swooning spells, close to blacks out or dazedness.

Other clinical issues that cause dazedness like heart beat issues.

Treatment

In the event that your PPPD is identified with another condition, similar to headache or nervousness, that condition ought to likewise be dealt with.

Exercise based recuperation

The sort of active recuperation used to treat PPPD is called adjustment treatment or openness treatment. This treatment opens you continuously to things that appear to cause your wooziness or aggravate it. The thought is that rehashed, brief openness to these things will assist you with developing a resilience to them, lessening your tipsiness.

You will have a treatment design and be approached to work through it at home.

It might require half a month to see critical improvement and no less than 8 to 12 weeks to get the best outcomes from your activity program.

Drugs

Two gatherings of drugs used to treat PPPD include:

Specific serotonin reuptake inhibitors, or SSRIs. These drugs are frequently used to treat discouragement and uneasiness yet appear to work in treating PPPD. Regardless of whether you are not discouraged or restless, SSRIs might assist with diminishing your discombobulation a ton.

Serotonin and norepinephrine reuptake inhibitors, or SNRIs. These meds are additionally used to treat gloom and nervousness. Regardless of whether you don't have a mental ailment, they can assist with diminishing your wooziness.

Step by step instructions to further develop balance

An individual can regularly work on their offset with home activities and active recuperation.

Work with a specialist or actual advisor to figure out which activities are protected, particularly if extreme dazedness is a successive issue.

When to see a specialist

It is ordinary to feel mixed up when wiped out, drained, smashed, or affected by specific drugs. Certain individuals additionally get tipsy when they are ravenous or restless.

Be that as it may, persistent equilibrium issues might show a genuine ailment. Brief analysis and treatment can further develop results and, sometimes, may even save lives.

See a specialist if an individual encounters:

• dizziness so extreme that they can't securely walk or drive

- dizziness that goes on for in excess of a couple of days

- periodic episodes of unsteadiness for reasons unknown

- other manifestations, like disarray

Go to the trauma centre if an individual encounters unsteadiness after a fall or auto collision, or then again in case there are indications of a stroke, like slurred discourse or deadness on one side of the body.

CHAPTER 3

REALITIES ABOUT PERSISTENT POSTURAL PERCEPTUAL DIZZINESS THAT ONE SHOULD KNOW

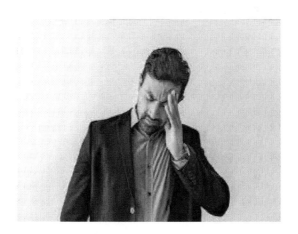

Feeling dazed and shaky can be perplexing, also risky when joined with security perils like a tricky floor. Be that as it may, for what reason does it occur in any case? Can an alignment specialist assist with dizziness and tipsiness? Do you have to manage these two manifestations your whole life? Justifiably, you may have a lot of inquiries stacking up in your mind as you can't help thinking about how to adapt better

when you experience a
scene. Is there an
opportunity to carry on with
an ordinary life?

How about we discover as
we take a gander at one of
the most exceedingly awful
incapacitating impacts of
ongoing dizziness assaults –
steady postural perceptual
wooziness or PPPD.

1. PPPD Leads to Certain Disturbances in One's Life

As its names recommend, PPPD or tireless postural perceptual unsteadiness can trigger repeating confounding scenes. At times, an assault can endure somewhere in the range of 24 hours to a few days. Other than confounding spells, it can cause the accompanying indications:

•	Feeling as though your body is drifting

•	Non-turning dizziness assaults (rather than seeing a turning sensation, your cerebrum believes you're encountering shaking or influencing developments)

•	Loss of equilibrium (you continually feel that

you will fall, excursion or slip at whatever point you move around)

Tragically, the PPPD manifestations can leave a significant effect on your timetable. It could keep you from working appropriately, particularly when the assault delays for a very long time.

2. PPPD Can Occasionally Affect Folks having Mood Disorders

A review clarifies that while jumble regularly emerges from vestibular issues, it can likewise get set off by a passionate ailment.

Not at all like in an ordinary condition, the cerebrum enters a touchy state when you have PPPD. That is the

reason you frequently dread
that you may slip or fall
each time a scene happens.

• 6 out of 10 patients
who have PPPD experience
mental episodes

• Only 25% of PPPD
patients don't report
disposition shifts

- About 45% of PPPD victims are clinically discouraged

3. PPPD Comes from Various Originating Conditions

When looking for replies to your inquiry, can a bone and joint specialist assist with dizziness and wooziness? This would assist you with tracking down the most reasonable way to deal with use. The following are the super fundamental medical conditions that regularly triggers the beginning of PPPD.

• Vestibular problems

Most cases, patients with Meniere's infection, different sclerosis, and harmless paroxysmal positional dizziness (BPPV), will in general become inclined to creating PPPD.

•   History of neck or head injury

A blackout or whiplash injury frequently brings about a neck misalignment that impacts your brainstem's typical capacity. It can likewise trigger a not insignificant rundown of vestibular issues like Meniere's and BPPV.

- Migraines

Approximately 4 out of 10 migraineurs likewise experience vestibular issues. On the off chance that you have ongoing vestibular headache scenes, you are likewise very liable to encounter PPPD side effects.

4. PPPD Diagnosis Can Be Tricky

Diagnosing vestibular issues are for the most part difficult to do. Additionally, relatively few individuals approach to have their side effects checked, so they never realize that their relentless bewildering spells and dizziness assaults really result from vestibular issues.

When diagnosing a suspected PPPD case, specialists need to direct a progression of tests to preclude other potential causes. First of all, you need to give subtleties on the recurrence and seriousness of your dizziness scenes. Then, at that point, you may have to go through different tests like adjusting tests and blood tests. At times the indicative strategy can require as long as 90 days or more, so you should be additionally patient.

5. Upper Cervical Care Provides Vertigo Relief

Upper cervical chiropractic might help in controlling the effect of your PPPD indications in your day to day existence. Basically, the methodology includes amending any primary issues with your C1 and C2 or upper cervical bones. These two sit under your skull as they support your head and take into consideration greatest developments. These two bones additionally secure your brainstem.

As a rule, patients who recently experienced neck and head wounds have neck bone misalignments. This triggers a chain of issues going from aggravation of the brainstem to the beginning of horrendous medical conditions, for example, dizziness assaults and even PPPD.

Accordingly, looking for upper cervical consideration may give you much-required alleviation from your PPPD side effects or other vestibular issues.

What Allows Greater Cervical Chiropractic Effective for PPPD Relief?

To be sure, having PPPD can give you many difficulties since it's a persistent type of vestibular problem. It could destroy an ideal day with your friends and family, influence your work efficiency levels and make you inclined to wounds and mishaps. Fortunately, you can take advantage of a characteristic solution via encountering less incessant and serious PPPD assaults.

Upper cervical consideration is a promising way to deal with vestibular problems like PPPD in light of the fact that it rectifies the issue's most probable reason – a skewed neck. The sooner you have your neck arrangement fixed. It will likewise re-establish your brainstem's typical capacity, permitting your body to recuperate from PPPD and its debilitating indications.

CHAPTER 4

SOME AMAZING THINGS THAT ONE NEEDS TO KNOW

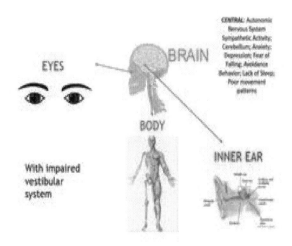

Ask your medical care

supplier any inquiries you

have about this data or about your tipsiness.

Discombobulated

Hazy headed

Substantial headed

Overcast headed

Cotton-headed

"Discombobulation" might be an inclination that your equilibrium is only not as great as it used to be. "Insecurity" alludes to a vibe of influencing or shaking that you get when you sit or stand. Insecurity may likewise be an impression of veering out of the way when strolling.

"Dizziness" is a sensation of turning or shifting unexpectedly. Dizziness isn't important for PPPD albeit certain individuals have PPPD alongside with different conditions that cause dizziness.

Constant postural-perceptual wooziness or PPPD is characterized as:

A sensation of discombobulation or flimsiness that you have more often than not

You have this sensation consistently.

This sensation has kept going no less than 90 days.

A few things might aggravate your PPPD:

Your own development

Development of things around you

Occupied stores

Parties

Traffic

"Outwardly requesting" things may likewise aggravate your PPPD. For instance:

Perusing

Dealing with the PC

Staring at the TV

Playing computer games

Strolling on floor coverings
with complex examples

PPPD can be identified with
different issues, or you can

have it without having any connected medical issues. Regardless, PPPD can be dealt with.

CHAPTER 5

HEALTH CARE TIPS PLUS SOME SALIENT QUESTIONS AND ANSWERS

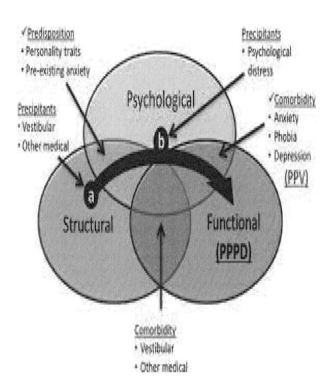

Accept your meds as recommended. Try not to quit taking them without conversing with your medical services supplier.

Things you can do:

Follow your treatment plan, including your home activities.

Accept your meds as your medical care supplier tells you to.

As you recuperate, find a steady speed. Enjoy reprieves from movement on a case by case basis.

Try not to restrict your exercises.

Every now and again ask questions

Is PPPD a mental ailment?

No, PPPD is certifiably not a mental problem. Yet, social changes can once in a while help. Thus, you might require seeing a medical doctor.

For what reason do I have PPPD?

We don't actually have the foggiest idea why individuals get PPPD. In the event that you had a connected condition, such as, an inward ear disease that gave you dizziness, you might have gotten touchier to your own development and equilibrium. This affectability might add to your PPPD.

Will I improve?

Around four out of five individuals seek better with treatment. Regardless of whether your unsteadiness doesn't disappear totally, treatment might help as time goes on.

How long do I require treatment?

Generally, the underlying time frame is from 8 to 12 weeks, for both exercise-based recuperation and drugs. Your treatment plan might keep going for a year or more.

Do the meds cause incidental effects?

SSRIs and the SNRIs might cause incidental effects. Get some information about conceivable incidental effects. You might see unsteadiness recorded as a potential result of these prescriptions. Nonetheless, that doesn't allude to the kind of tipsiness brought about by PPPD. Once in a while PPPD is aggravated by SSRIs or SNRIs.

How might I be certain that PPPD is what I have?

Proper medical examinations by your doctor will reveal to you that you have PPPD.

CHAPTER6

CONCLUSION

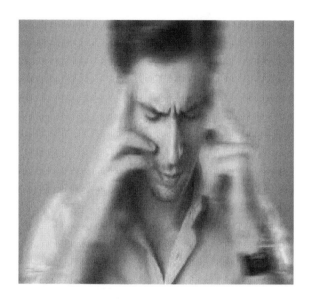

Certain individuals might discover discombobulation alarming, and it can influence their personal satisfaction. Much of the time, it is feasible to get the real reason or take out manifestations of dazedness.

On the off chance that an individual has worries about tipsiness, they should converse with a specialist or doctor.

THE END.

Manufactured by Amazon.ca
Bolton, ON

38034823R00042